MOXIBUSTION FOR BEGINNERS

Comprehensive Guide To Techniques, Benefits For Optimal Health And Wellness

DR SAWYER DIEGO

DISCLAMER

Nothing in this book should be interpreted as medical advice; it is meant exclusively for educational reasons. Regarding their specific health issues and treatment options, readers are urged to speak with licensed healthcare professionals. The publisher and author disclaim all liability for any errors or omissions in the material provided, as well as for any negative effects that may arise from using or abusing the information. Although every attempt has been taken to guarantee that the material in this book is correct as of the date of publishing, new research may have superseded some of the content because medical knowledge is always changing. It is recommended that readers confirm the most recent medical recommendations and guidelines. The reader of this book undertakes to release the author and publisher from any claims or liabilities resulting from the use of this information, and understands and accepts the inherent risks connected with healthcare decisions.

TABLE OF CONTENTS

ABOUT THE BOOK

"Moxibustion for Beginners" provides a thorough overview of the fundamentals and advantages of moxibustion, making it a valuable resource for both novices and experts looking to expand their knowledge of this age-old therapeutic technique with roots in traditional Chinese medicine.

The book starts by explaining what moxibustion is and how it works in conjunction with acupuncture to promote holistic wellness. It then goes into detail about the historical roots of moxibustion and how it has developed over centuries, clarifying important terms and ideas that are essential to its practice. Safety is covered in detail so that readers are aware of the precautions and contraindications, which are especially important when incorporating moxibustion into regular healthcare routines.

The book begins with a thorough examination of moxibustion techniques, outlining the differences between direct and indirect methods as well as discussing smokeless options and moxa material selection. It then goes on to provide readers with helpful advice on how to set up a safe and conducive environment and select appropriate acupuncture points, preparing them for safe and successful therapy sessions. Finally, the book concludes with an integration of aromatherapy and relaxation techniques that improve therapeutic outcomes and patient comfort during treatments.

The advantages and therapeutic qualities of moxibustion are thoroughly reviewed, emphasizing its effectiveness in reducing pain, enhancing circulation, boosting immunity, and addressing a range of digestive and emotional health issues. Frequently asked questions, including possible adverse effects, safety for particular populations, such as children and pregnant women, and methods to lessen discomfort, is carefully considered, guaranteeing a comprehensive approach to wellness.

FAQs help readers understand moxibustion by answering questions about safety, applications, and acupuncture integration. Practical advice covers how to incorporate moxibustion into daily wellness routines and encourages readers to customize schedules and consult a professional to monitor progress. Advanced applications discuss moxibustion's role in sports medicine, rehabilitation, and chronic pain management, highlighting ongoing research and new developments in therapy and equipment.

"Moxibustion for Beginners" is a gateway to a time-honored practice, offering both practical guidance and a profound journey into holistic health and wellness. Finally, the book looks toward the future of moxibustion, highlighting innovations, sustainability in materials, and educational resources. It invites readers to explore cultural and spiritual dimensions, fostering a deeper appreciation and engagement with this ancient healing art.

CHAPTER ONE
MOXIBUSTION OVERVIEW
MOXIBUSTION DEFINITION

Moxibustion is an age-old traditional Chinese medicine (TCM) technique that involves burning mugwort (Artemisia vulgaris) to stimulate acupuncture points on the body. The goal of this therapeutic technique is to improve the flow of Qi (vital energy) through the meridians, promoting health and balance. There are two main types of moxibustion: indirect and direct. In indirect moxibustion, a moxa stick is held above the skin without touching it, producing a softer heat.

Choosing the right acupuncture points based on the patient's condition and TCM diagnosis is the first step in the moxibustion process. The practitioner then cleans the area and may apply a protective ointment to minimize any potential discomfort or skin irritation. After lighting the moxa, the heat it produces permeates the acupuncture point, stimulating circulation and Qi flow, which is thought to relieve pain, reduce inflammation, and boost immunity. The moxa ash is disposed of safely at the end of the session, and any lingering heat feeling usually goes away quickly.

A beginner to moxibustion should consult with qualified practitioners to ensure safe and effective treatment, as proper training and knowledge of acupuncture points are crucial for its therapeutic benefits. Moxibustion's application varies depending on the condition being treated, ranging from chronic pain management to digestive disorders and fertility issues. Understanding moxibustion involves appreciating its role within the broader framework of traditional Chinese medicine, where it is often used in conjunction with acupuncture and herbal medicine.

ADVANTAGES OF MOXIBUSTION TREATMENT

Due to its capacity to stimulate Qi and support the body's inherent healing processes, moxibustion therapy has several potential advantages. The first is that it can effectively relieve pain, especially in cases of arthritis, muscle strain, and menstrual cramps. Additionally, by warming the meridians and improving blood circulation, moxibustion can help reduce inflammation and improve joint mobility, making it an invaluable adjunctive therapy for chronic pain management and rehabilitation.

Additionally, moxibustion is well-known for strengthening immunity, which makes it advantageous for people with compromised immune systems or during cold and flu seasons. The heat produced by moxa stimulates the production of white blood cells and improves immune function in general, helping to prevent illness and hasten recovery. Furthermore, moxibustion is frequently used to support digestive health by regulating gastrointestinal function and easing symptoms of bloating, indigestion, and irritable bowel syndrome.

As a non-invasive therapy, moxibustion is generally well-tolerated with minimal side effects when administered correctly; however, individuals with sensitive skin or specific health conditions should seek guidance from a qualified practitioner to ensure safe and effective treatment catered to their needs. From a holistic standpoint, moxibustion not only targets specific ailments but also promotes overall well-being by balancing the body's energy flow.

THE ORIGINS AND HISTORY OF MOXIBUSTION

The origins of moxibustion can be traced back thousands of years to ancient China, where it developed alongside acupuncture and herbal medicine as essential components of traditional Chinese medicine (TCM).

Moxibustion was first used to treat a variety of illnesses and promote general health during the Han Dynasty (206 BCE–220 CE). Over the centuries, moxibustion techniques evolved to reflect regional variations and advances in medical knowledge.

The foundation of moxibustion in traditional Chinese medicine is the idea of preserving harmony and balance within the body's energy systems, or Qi. Diseases were thought to arise from disturbances or obstructions in the flow of Qi along meridians, and moxibustion was used to restore this flow and promote healing. As TCM spread outside of China, moxibustion became well-liked in other East Asian nations like Japan and Korea, where it was incorporated into their respective medical traditions.

Moxibustion has been used for millennia because mugwort (Artemisia vulgaris) has therapeutic qualities and burns evenly without emitting a lot of smoke. Different techniques were developed, such as direct and indirect moxibustion, which allowed practitioners to customize treatments to the needs of individual patients while reducing potential discomfort or side effects. Moxibustion is still used today in traditional medical settings and is becoming more and more integrated into complementary and alternative medicine practices around the world.

Its durability and extensive adoption highlight its efficacy in treating a range of diseases and its continued significance in holistic health practices. An understanding of the historical background of moxibustion offers insights into its enduring relevance and evolution as a therapeutic modality.

RECOGNIZING IMPORTANT WORDS AND IDEAS

Understanding key terms and concepts that are fundamental to the practice of moxibustion within traditional Chinese medicine (TCM) is imperative to fully comprehend the art of moxibustion. At the core of moxibustion is the concept of Qi, which is often translated as vital energy or life force. TCM principles hold that Qi flows through the body along specific pathways called meridians, influencing general health and well-being.

Moxibustion seeks to regulate this flow of Qi, addressing imbalances that materialize as illness or discomfort.

The key component of moxibustion therapy is the use of acupuncture points or acupoints. These are specific locations along the meridians where Qi can be accessed and manipulated, chosen based on TCM diagnosis. By applying moxibustion to these acupoints, practitioners stimulate Qi circulation, encourage blood flow, and relieve symptoms related to a variety of health conditions.

The use of mugwort (Artemisia vulgaris), a herb known for its therapeutic properties, is another key idea in moxibustion. Dried mugwort leaves are processed into various forms, such as sticks, cones, or loose fibers, which are then burned. The heat produced by burning moxa is thought to permeate deeply into tissues, warming the acupoints and promoting the flow of Qi. This application of therapeutic heat sets moxibustion apart from other forms of heat therapy and emphasizes its special advantages in traditional Chinese medicine.

Knowing these basic terms and concepts helps beginners better understand and appreciate the therapeutic principles of moxibustion. Understanding the connections between Qi, meridians, acupoints, and moxa emphasizes the holistic nature of moxibustion and how it fits into more comprehensive treatment plans in traditional Chinese medicine.

SAFETY OBSERVATIONS AND SAFETY MEASURES

The risk of burns is the main concern with moxibustion, especially with direct methods where the moxa comes into direct contact with the skin. Practitioners should exercise caution to avoid excessive heat exposure and monitor the patient's comfort level throughout the session.

Protective measures like applying a barrier cream or using a protective layer between the skin and moxa can help mitigate this risk. Even though moxibustion is generally considered safe and well-tolerated, it is essential to observe certain safety considerations and precautions to ensure optimal outcomes and minimize potential risks.

A safe and comfortable treatment experience is dependent on practitioners educating patients about potential smoke exposure and addressing any concerns they may have. Moreover, the smoke produced during moxibustion can cause respiratory difficulties, particularly for those who have asthma or sensitivity to smoke. Sufficient ventilation in the treatment area is essential to dissipate smoke and minimize exposure. Practitioners may choose to use smokeless moxa preparations or indirect moxibustion methods, which produce less smoke while still delivering therapeutic benefits.

Proper disposal of moxa ash and cleaning of treatment surfaces contribute to a hygienic environment conducive to healing. Hygiene practices are also crucial during moxibustion sessions to prevent infection and maintain cleanliness. Practitioners should sanitize their hands before and after treatment and ensure sterile handling of moxa materials. Disposable or single-use moxa products can further reduce the risk of contamination.

Individual health concerns should direct the application of moxibustion, especially for women who are pregnant, people with skin conditions, or people undergoing medical treatments. It is crucial for safety and efficacy to seek the advice of a qualified practitioner who can evaluate each patient's health status and customize moxibustion treatment accordingly. By following these safety guidelines and precautions, practitioners and patients can safely integrate moxibustion into their wellness routines, utilizing its therapeutic benefits while guaranteeing a comfortable and safe experience.

CHAPTER TWO
UNDERSTANDING MOXIBUSTION
SYNOPSIS OF MOXIBUSTION TREATMENT

A fundamental component of traditional Chinese medicine (TCM), moxibustion therapy involves burning mugwort (Artemisia vulgaris) to stimulate acupuncture points on the body. The goal of this therapy is to enhance the flow of Qi, the vital energy believed to flow through pathways (meridians) in the body. Practitioners choose which points to burn depending on the patient's condition and treatment objectives. There are two types of moxibustion: indirect and direct. Indirect moxibustion uses a moxa stick held above the skin or placed on acupuncture needles to heat the area without direct contact.

As a preventive measure to maintain wellness and balance in the body, practitioners of TCM theory use moxibustion to dispel cold and dampness, promote circulation, and enhance overall health. Moxibustion is frequently used to treat conditions like chronic pain, digestive disorders, and irregular menstruation, and to boost the immune system. Practitioners who comprehend the principles underlying moxibustion can apply this therapy effectively, utilizing heat and herbs to support health and well-being.

MOXIBUSTION AND ACUPUNCTURE DISTINCTIONS

Although moxibustion and acupuncture are essential components of Traditional Chinese Medicine (TCM), they are not the same in application or therapeutic emphasis. While acupuncture uses thin needles inserted into specific body points to promote Qi flow and healing, moxibustion primarily uses heat from burning mugwort to warm and stimulate acupuncture points. TCM uses acupuncture to treat a wide range of conditions, from emotional disorders to pain management, by manipulating the flow of Qi along meridians. Moxibustion, on the other hand, focuses on warming and tonifying the body, especially useful for ailments associated with cold or deficiency.

Understanding these differences helps practitioners tailor treatments to individual patient needs, choosing the most appropriate therapy or combination based on the diagnosis and health goals. By integrating moxibustion and acupuncture, practitioners can offer comprehensive TCM treatments that effectively address a wide range of health concerns. Both therapies can be used independently or in combination to enhance treatment efficacy. Acupuncture needles may be heated with moxa during treatment (moxa acupuncture).

HEAT AND HERBS ARE IMPORTANT IN TRADITIONAL CHINESE MEDICINE

Traditional Chinese medicine (TCM) places great emphasis on the therapeutic application of heat and herbs. TCM theory holds that heat stimulates circulation, drives away cold and dampness, and facilitates the flow of Qi and blood. Through the application of heat to acupuncture points, practitioners hope to enhance the body's natural healing capabilities and bring about a state of balance. The herb used in moxibustion, mugwort, is chosen for its warming qualities and capacity to tonify Qi. The combination of heat and herbs in moxibustion supports several health benefits, such as pain relief, immune support, and digestive regulation.

The use of heat and herbs in TCM reflects a holistic approach to health, emphasizing the interconnectedness of the body, mind, and environment. By understanding the importance of heat and herbs in moxibustion, practitioners can optimize treatment outcomes and support patients in achieving long-term health goals.

Herbal medicine in TCM encompasses a vast array of plants and minerals used to address specific health conditions and promote overall well-being. When used in moxibustion, mugwort is carefully selected and prepared to maximize its therapeutic effects.

FREQUENTLY HELD MYTHS REGARDING MOXIBUSTION

In modern contexts, moxibustion therapy is still widely misunderstood despite its long history and therapeutic benefits. First, it is a common misconception that moxibustion involves burning the skin directly; in fact, practitioners take care to prevent burns by closely monitoring the application of heat in both direct and indirect moxibustion techniques. Secondly, patients often report feeling relaxed and soothed after a moxibustion session, often describing gentle warmth at the treatment site.

Additionally, some people might think that moxibustion is just superstitious or based on tradition rather than science. Nevertheless, studies on the physiological effects of moxibustion show that it can regulate immune responses, improve circulation, and decrease inflammation. Dispelling these myths enables both patients and practitioners to recognize moxibustion as an effective therapeutic modality within the larger context of traditional Chinese medicine. After learning about the fundamentals of moxibustion, people can decide whether or not to incorporate it into their daily routines.

THE ADVANTAGES OF INCLUDING MOXIBUSTION IN WELLNESS PRACTICES

Including moxibustion in wellness regimens have many advantages for general health and vitality. Firstly, it can boost immunity by improving circulation and Qi flow, which can help the body fend against illness and heal from common ailments more quickly. Secondly, moxibustion is beneficial for pain relief, especially chronic pain from conditions like arthritis or muscle strain.

By warming certain acupuncture points, moxibustion can reduce inflammation and increase joint mobility.

The promotion of digestive health is another important advantage of moxibustion. It can help with indigestion, bloating, and irregular bowel movements by stimulating the digestive organs and regulating Qi flow. Many people find that adding moxibustion to their wellness routines helps them relax and de-stress. The mild warmth of moxibustion sessions can have a calming effect on the nervous system, supporting mental and emotional well-being.

Since moxibustion supports the body's natural healing processes and improves overall quality of life, its benefits go beyond symptomatic relief and include holistic health maintenance and prevention. Knowing these benefits encourages people to investigate moxibustion as a complementary therapy in addition to traditional medical treatments, thereby promoting comprehensive health and well-being.

CHAPTER THREE
MANY MOXIBUSTION TYPES
METHODS OF MOXIBUSTION: DIRECT VERSUS INDIRECT

There are two main methods used in moxibustion therapy: direct and indirect. Direct moxibustion is applying moxa directly to the skin or over an acupuncture needle inserted into the skin. The heat from burning the moxa penetrates deeply into the acupuncture point, causing circulation to increase and healing to occur. This method is often used for conditions that require deep penetration of heat or strong stimulation. It is important to watch the burning moxa closely during the session to prevent burns or discomfort.

Indirect moxibustion, on the other hand, is a safer alternative in which the moxa is not in direct contact with the skin. To moderate the heat, practitioners usually place a layer of insulation, such as ginger, salt, or a slice of garlic, between the moxa and the skin.

This method is gentler and appropriate for people who are new to moxibustion therapy or have sensitive skin. Despite the low risk of burns, indirect moxibustion still enhances qi circulation and warms the acupuncture point, providing therapeutic benefits. Beginners can learn this technique more easily with the right guidance to ensure safe and effective treatment outcomes.

Direct and indirect moxibustion each have specific advantages and safety precautions that make them useful tools in traditional Chinese medicine for promoting health and wellness. By learning these techniques, beginners can select the best approach based on the condition being treated and personal preferences.

RECOGNIZING YOUR OPTIONS FOR SMOKELESS MOXIBUSTION

For those who prefer the benefits of moxibustion without the inconvenience of lingering odors or respiratory discomfort, smokeless moxibustion offers a viable alternative. Smokeless moxibustion addresses concerns about traditional moxa's smoke and odor, providing a cleaner and more comfortable experience for both practitioners and clients. This technique involves specially processed moxa that reduces smoke production while retaining its therapeutic properties.

Selecting the best option for smokeless moxibustion entails taking into account various aspects, including the kind of processing employed the moxa's material composition, and the desired therapeutic result. Certain products for smokeless moxibustion minimize smoke emission while maximizing the moxibustion effect; novices investigating this technique should make sure they buy high-quality smokeless moxa from reliable vendors to guarantee safety and effectiveness in their practice.

Correct application of smokeless moxibustion maximizes its therapeutic benefits while fostering a comfortable treatment environment.

With the availability of smokeless moxibustion options, practitioners can meet health and safety regulations for moxibustion practice while still providing improved treatment experiences. These options satisfy contemporary preferences for cleaner therapies without sacrificing the efficacy of traditional moxibustion techniques.

SELECTING THE APPROPRIATE MOXA MATERIALS

To ensure that moxibustion therapy is as effective as possible, beginners need to choose high-quality rolls or cones produced under controlled conditions to ensure purity and efficacy in therapy. Traditional moxa is typically made from mugwort (Artemisia vulgaris) leaves, which contain essential oils and other active compounds believed to enhance therapeutic effects. The potency and consistency of the mugwort in heat generation during moxibustion are determined by the quality and processing method of the mugwort.

In addition, practitioners can select smokeless moxa options made of charcoal or herbal additives, which provide a cleaner burning and less smoke emission than traditional moxa. These alternatives can be customized to meet the needs of individual clients and address particular health issues, making them flexible options in moxibustion practice. Knowledge of the characteristics and uses of various moxa materials helps novices customize treatment plans to meet the needs of each patient while guaranteeing safe and efficient therapeutic results.

By investigating different types of moxa materials, practitioners can be more adaptable in tailoring moxibustion therapy to a wide range of client needs and medical conditions.

HOW DIFFERENT TECHNIQUES AFFECT HEAT INTENSITY

It is important for beginners to carefully control the duration and distance of the Moxa application to prevent overheating and ensure client comfort during treatment. The intensity of heat in moxibustion therapy varies depending on the technique used and the specific conditions being treated. Direct moxibustion techniques typically generate higher heat intensity due to direct contact between the burning moxa and the skin or acupuncture point. This method allows for deeper penetration of heat, making it suitable for conditions requiring strong stimulation or pain relief.

Understanding how heat intensity varies between moxibustion techniques allows practitioners to tailor treatments according to individual preferences and health conditions. In contrast, indirect moxibustion techniques moderate heat intensity by placing insulation materials between the moxa and the skin. This method lowers the risk of burns while still providing therapeutic warmth to the acupuncture point, and beginners can adjust the amount and thickness of insulation based on client sensitivity and treatment goals to achieve optimal therapeutic outcomes without discomfort.

While retaining the therapeutic benefits of traditional moxibustion, the incorporation of smokeless moxibustion options further refines heat intensity control by providing cleaner combustion and increased comfort during therapy. Practitioners can be more flexible in adjusting heat levels with these alternatives and by learning the variations in heat intensity in moxibustion techniques, novices can safely and effectively treat each client according to their individual needs and preferences.

ADVICE ON SAFETY FOR EVERY KIND OF MOXIBUSTION

To avoid burns or unfavorable reactions, safety during moxibustion therapy is crucial. When using direct moxibustion, practitioners should watch the burning moxa carefully and adjust its position to avoid prolonged skin contact. Protective barriers like ginger slices or salt can help regulate heat and reduce the risk of burns, especially in sensitive areas or with clients who are prone to skin irritation.

To minimize the risk of burns, beginners should inform clients about the feeling of warmth they may experience.

To maintain safe heat levels during indirect moxibustion, practitioners must carefully choose and apply the insulation materials; they must also regularly assess skin condition and client feedback to prevent overheating and ensure a positive treatment experience; and they must ensure that smokeless moxa options reduce smoke exposure and enhance treatment safety for both practitioners and clients, thereby fostering a supportive environment for moxibustion therapy.

By putting client safety and comfort first, novices can establish credibility and trust in their moxibustion practice while producing successful therapeutic results. The implementation of thorough safety protocols and ongoing training also increases practitioners' confidence and skill in moxibustion techniques.

CHAPTER FOUR

GETTING READY FOR MOXIBUSTION

CREATING A SECURE AND COZY ENVIRONMENT

For a moxibustion session to be successful, the following conditions must be met: the room must be peaceful, well-ventilated, and quiet so that you can relax undisturbed; it should also be comfortably warm to maximize the therapeutic effects of moxibustion; clutter must be removed; and the recipient must have a comfortable surface to lie on, such as a massage table or padded mat.

A calm and safe environment is necessary to maximize the benefits of moxibustion therapy. To further enhance safety, remove any flammable materials from the area and keep a fire extinguisher nearby as a precaution.

Soft lighting or ambient lighting can help create a calming atmosphere conducive to relaxation. You may want to play soft music or nature sounds to promote relaxation during the session.

GETTING THE SUPPLIES AND EQUIPMENT NEEDED

To guarantee a seamless and uninterrupted moxibustion session, make sure you have all the tools and supplies you'll need before you start. These include premium moxa sticks or cones, a moxa extinguisher or bowl of sand for securely extinguishing moxa, a lighter or matches for lighting the moxa, and cotton wool or a protective cream to shield the recipient's skin from direct heat.

Depending on the type of moxibustion you choose—direct or indirect—you may also need special tools like moxa boxes, acupuncture needles, or bamboo holders to securely hold the burning moxa in place over the acupuncture points. Having all supplies organized and within reach helps maintain the flow of the session and ensures a professional approach to moxibustion therapy.

Additionally, have clean towels or blankets on hand to cover the recipient and keep them warm during and after the session.

METHODS FOR CHOOSING THE CORRECT ACUPUNCTURE POINTS

Selecting the appropriate acupuncture points is essential to successful moxibustion treatment. Become familiar with the meridian system and the particular points linked to the ailment or symptoms you plan to treat. Points linked to pain management, immune system stimulation, and overall healths are frequently used for moxibustion.

Accurate location of these points can be achieved by consulting acupuncture charts or guides. Feeling the area gently will reveal any tenderness or sensitivity, which is often a sign of an active acupuncture point. For novices, familiar and easily accessible points such as LI4 (Hegu) for pain relief or ST36 (Zusanli) for energy enhancement can offer a useful introduction to moxibustion therapy.

Knowledge of the principles governing acupuncture point selection guarantees focused and successful treatment outcomes.

GETTING THE SKIN READY FOR MOXIBUSTION TREATMENT

For both safety and efficacy, the skin must be properly prepared before applying moxibustion. To start, wash the skin well with mild soap and water to get rid of any residue from lotions, oils, or dirt. Next, pat dry the skin with a clean towel to make sure it is completely dry before continuing. If needed, shave any extra hair from the area to prevent burning or discomfort during the moxibustion session.

Before beginning moxibustion therapy, make sure the recipient is comfortable and relaxed. A relaxed state leads to better therapeutic outcomes. Apply a thin layer of protective cream or petroleum jelly around the acupuncture point to shield the surrounding skin from direct heat. This protects the skin and also makes the moxa stick or cone easier to move.

INCLUDING AROMATHERAPY AND CALMING METHODS

Aromatherapy and relaxation techniques can be used to enhance the therapeutic benefits of moxibustion. Select essential oils that are known for their calming or invigorating qualities, such as peppermint for mental clarity or lavender for relaxation. Apply a few drops of the chosen oil to pulse points or diffuse it throughout the room using an essential oil diffuser.

Aromatherapy combined with moxibustion not only relaxes the mind and body but also enhances the overall therapeutic experience. Encourage deep breathing exercises or guided relaxation techniques to help the recipient achieve a state of deep relaxation during moxibustion.

Lightly massage or acupressure on non-treated areas can further promote relaxation and enhance the overall therapeutic experience.

To conduct safe and successful moxibustion therapy sessions, it is imperative that a harmonious environment be created and that thorough preparation be made. By adhering to these doable rules and strategies, novices can confidently perform moxibustion therapy, fostering balance and wellness in both themselves and their clients.

CHAPTER FIVE

METHODS FOR MOXIBUSTION IN STEPS

COMPREHENSIVE GUIDE TO DIRECT MOXIBUSTION TECHNIQUES

A classic therapeutic method, direct moxibustion applies ignited moxa directly to the skin at predetermined acupuncture points. To perform direct moxibustion, collect your materials (tweezers, moxa cones or sticks, and a heat-resistant base, like a small plate or slice of ginger). Select the acupuncture points according to your treatment objectives and make sure the patient is at ease and aware of the procedure.

First, light the moxa stick with tweezers and hold it there until it forms a glowing ember. Then, carefully place the moxa stick onto the chosen acupuncture point, making sure it's close but not touching the skin directly.

The heat should gently penetrate to stimulate the point. Throughout the procedure, keep an eye on the patient's comfort level and adjust the moxa stick's distance if needed.

After the session is over, safely extinguish the moxa stick and give the patient aftercare instructions. When done correctly and safely, direct moxibustion can improve circulation, relieve pain, and promote general well-being. The recommended duration of each point is usually ten to fifteen minutes.

DETAILED GUIDELINES FOR INDIRECT MOXIBUSTION

Select appropriate acupuncture points, make sure the patient is comfortable and relaxed, prepare the treatment area, explain the procedure to them, and then apply a moxa stick or cone indirectly on the acupuncture points. A barrier, such as ginger slices or salt, is often placed between the moxa and the skin to moderate the heat intensity.

Position the moxa above the barrier and adjust the distance based on the patient's comfort and therapeutic goals.

Light the moxa stick or cone until it forms a glowing ember. Hold it close to the skin, but not touching it. Protect the skin from direct heat by placing a slice of ginger or a small amount of salt on the acupuncture point.

When the session is over, safely extinguish the moxa and give instructions for post-treatment care. When used carefully and meticulously, indirect moxibustion can effectively tonify qi, strengthen yang energy, and promote relaxation.

Let the moxa burn and warm the area for 10–20 minutes per point, monitoring the patient's response throughout.

ENHANCING THERAPY WITH STICKS AND ROLLS OF MOXA

Compressed moxa rolls and sticks, which come in a variety of sizes and shapes (e.g., cigar-shaped moxa sticks or moxa rolls with high-quality moxa herbs compressed into convenient forms for direct or indirect application), are useful tools used in traditional moxibustion therapies to enhance therapeutic effects.

For direct moxibustion, place the moxa stick directly onto the acupuncture point or area of treatment, adjusting the heat intensity as necessary. To use moxa rolls or sticks, choose the right size and shape according to the treatment area and desired therapeutic effect. Light the moxa and let it form a smoldering ember.

To get the appropriate therapeutic effect, position the moxa roll above the barrier and vary the distance to achieve it. For indirect moxibustion, use moxa rolls with a barrier, such as ginger slices, to moderate heat. Closely monitor the treatment process, making sure the patient is comfortable and safe at all times.

When used correctly in moxibustion therapy, moxa rolls and sticks can improve circulation, reduce pain, and aid in healing. They provide practitioners with flexibility in application methods while preserving the potency of moxa herbs for overall health benefits.

MODIFYING TEMPERATURE IN MOXIBUSTION SESSIONS

Heat intensity can be moderated depending on the type of moxibustion—direct or indirect—and the sensitivity of the acupuncture points being treated. Appropriate adjustment maximizes therapeutic benefits while minimizing discomfort or risk of burns. Adjusting heat levels during moxibustion sessions is essential to ensuring effective treatment outcomes and patient comfort.

While performing direct moxibustion, keep a close eye on the glowing ember of the moxa stick or cone. Modify the distance between the moxa and the skin to regulate the amount of heat—closer proximity results in more heat, greater distance results in less heat—and pay attention to the patient's feedback to maintain a therapeutic but comfortable temperature.

Use barriers such as salt or ginger slices to moderate heat transmission to the skin when using indirect moxibustion; if the patient feels uncomfortable, place extra layers or move the moxa to a different location. Throughout the session, keep an eye out for any signs of skin sensitivity or overheating in the treatment area to ensure safety and efficacy.

Practitioners can effectively optimize moxibustion therapy to stimulate acupuncture points, improve circulation, and promote overall wellness by adjusting heat levels skillfully. Achieving proficiency in this crucial area of traditional Chinese medicine requires regular practice and sensitivity to patient responses.

COMBINING TRADITIONAL THERAPIES WITH MOXIBUSTION

Integrating moxibustion with acupuncture, herbal medicine, or massage therapy offers holistic benefits by addressing both symptoms and underlying imbalances in the body.

Combining moxibustion with other traditional therapies can improve treatment outcomes and address a variety of health concerns synergistically.

For example, when combining moxibustion and acupuncture, choose your acupuncture points according to traditional meridian theory and treatment objectives. Apply moxibustion either before or following acupuncture needling to strengthen therapeutic effects and improve qi circulation. Depending on the patient's condition, this combination can reduce pain, promote better digestion, and strengthen immunity.

When combining moxibustion with herbal medicine, use warming herbs to enhance the warming effects of moxa. Make herbal concoctions that nourish the blood, expel cold, or tonify qi, which will improve moxibustion's ability to regulate body functions and heal. Treatment plans should be coordinated with herbalists or practitioners of traditional Chinese medicine for all-encompassing care.

Warming particular meridians or muscle groups can help release tension and encourage relaxation. Indirect moxibustion techniques, such as using moxa rolls, can be used to target areas of imbalance or stagnation found during massage assessments. Treatments should be tailored to the patient's constitution and therapeutic goals for best outcomes.

Incorporating moxibustion with other conventional therapies allows practitioners to provide patients with comprehensive care that attends to the physical, emotional, and spiritual aspects of health. Individual treatment plans can be customized, and multidisciplinary teams can work together to optimize therapeutic outcomes and advance overall health.

CHAPTER SIX

ADVANTAGES AND RESTORATIVE QUALITIES

EXAMINING MOXIBUSTION'S THERAPEUTIC EFFECTS

An ancient Chinese therapy called moxibustion uses the power of burning dried mugwort, or moxa, near specific acupuncture points on the body to promote energy flow (Qi) and balance the body. By applying heat to these points, moxibustion improves circulation, eases tension in the muscles and joints, and promotes relaxation.

Moxibustion is frequently combined with acupuncture to enhance its therapeutic effects and offer a comprehensive approach to health and well-being.

It is thought to activate the body's natural healing mechanisms, facilitating the release of endorphins and reducing inflammation. The warmth generated during moxibustion penetrates deeply into tissues, promoting healing and alleviating conditions such as chronic pain, arthritis, and menstrual cramps. Practitioners frequently customize treatments based on the individual's specific health needs, targeting areas where energy stagnation or deficiency is detected through traditional diagnostic methods.

Frequent sessions of moxibustion are advised for the prevention and maintenance of general health. Its mild yet profound effect on the body's energy pathways makes it appropriate for a variety of conditions, from respiratory ailments to musculoskeletal disorders.

Moxibustion is a non-invasive therapy that provides a natural solution for individuals seeking relief from chronic health issues while fostering a sense of relaxation and well-being.

APPLICATIONS FOR THE MANAGEMENT AND RELIEF OF PAIN

The use of moxibustion goes beyond treating acute pain to include managing chronic pain as well.

Moxibustion works by focusing on specific acupuncture points that correspond with pain pathways, which lessens the intensity and frequency of pain. It is especially useful for treating conditions like neuropathic pain, migraines, and lower back pain, for which traditional treatments may provide only patchy relief.

Burning moxa increases circulation and triggers the body to release endorphins, which are naturally occurring chemicals that reduce pain. This combined effect not only reduces pain but also speeds up the healing and recovery process. Moxibustion is frequently included in treatment plans in conjunction with acupuncture and other complementary therapies to improve patient outcomes and quality of life for those with chronic pain.

Following regular sessions, patients report notable increases in mobility and decreased dependency on painkillers. Moxibustion's targeted approach enables practitioners to customize treatments according to each patient's unique pain patterns and health conditions, guaranteeing individualized care that targets the underlying causes of pain rather than just masking its symptoms. Moxibustion is a safe, non-invasive therapy that presents a promising alternative for those looking for natural pain relief options without unfavorable side effects.

INCREASING IMMUNE RESPONSE AND CIRCULATION

Moxibustion is a valuable therapy for promoting overall health and vitality because of its ability to improve circulation and enhance immune function. It also helps to remove metabolic waste products, reduce inflammation, and speed up the body's healing responses by stimulating blood flow to targeted areas, which helps to deliver oxygen and nutrients to tissues more efficiently and supports cellular repair and regeneration.

Frequent use of moxibustion sessions has been demonstrated to boost immunity by stimulating immune cells and improving their capacity to fight pathogens and foreign invaders. This immune-boosting effect is especially advantageous for those who are prone to infections or are recuperating from illness. The mild yet effective effects of moxibustion on immune function highlight the practice's potential as a preventive therapy for preserving health and resilience against seasonal health challenges.

Apart from its physical advantages, moxibustion also contributes to emotional and mental health because it can balance Qi, or energy flow, throughout the body. It also lowers stress and anxiety levels by promoting calmness and relaxation through the harmonization of the body's internal systems.

UTILIZING MOXIBUSTION TO TREAT DIGESTIVE DISORDERS

Moxibustion therapy is a promising treatment for a variety of digestive disorders, from simple dyspepsia to more complicated conditions like gastritis and irritable bowel syndrome (IBS). Moxibustion works by focusing on specific digestive acupuncture points to help regulate gastrointestinal function, relieve symptoms like bloating and discomfort, and enhance overall digestive efficiency.

Moxibustion is frequently incorporated into comprehensive treatment plans alongside dietary adjustments and lifestyle modifications to support long-term digestive health. The heat generated by burning moxa stimulates peristalsis, the wave-like contractions of the digestive tract that propel food through the stomach and intestines. This action helps to relieve stagnation and promote smoother digestion, reducing symptoms of acid reflux, constipation, and abdominal pain.

In addition to its gentle yet effective approach, moxibustion is appropriate for people of all ages seeking natural alternatives to manage chronic digestive conditions without solely relying on medications. Patients who undergo moxibustion for digestive issues often report improvements in appetite, regularity of bowel movements, and a reduction in gastrointestinal discomfort.

Moxibustion's restoration of digestive system balance also contributes to overall health and vitality, fostering a sense of well-being and improved quality of life.

HANDLING ANXIETY, STRESS, AND EMOTIONAL WELL-BEING

Targeting specific acupuncture points associated with the nervous system and emotional centers of the brain, moxibustion offers a holistic approach to managing stress, anxiety, and emotional health in addition to physical ailments. It also helps to regulate mood, lower anxiety levels, and foster a sense of relaxation and inner calm.

Moxibustion is frequently recommended for those experiencing symptoms of anxiety disorders, depression, and mood swings as part of a comprehensive treatment plan because the heat generated during the procedure stimulates the release of endorphins and other neurotransmitters that promote feelings of happiness and well-being.

This naturally occurring mood-enhancing effect can help individuals cope with daily stressors more effectively, improving resilience and emotional stability.

Frequent moxibustion sessions support the mind-body connection and help the body's energy flow (Qi) to remain in balance. This integrative approach to emotional health highlights the connection between physical and mental health and provides patients with a natural, non-invasive alternative to traditional therapies. Moxibustion also fosters emotional resilience and overall vitality, which extends beyond symptom management to quality of life and long-term health outcomes.

CHAPTER SEVEN

TYPICAL ISSUES AND SAFETY FACTORS

POSSIBLE ADVERSE REACTIONS AND SAFETY MEASURES

As with any therapy, moxibustion carries some risk and needs to be used with caution. Common side effects include localized skin irritation or burns from direct contact with the burning moxa or from excessive heat exposure. It is important to use moxibustion under the supervision of a trained practitioner to minimize these risks.

Moxibustion is a traditional Chinese medicine practice that involves burning dried mugwort (moxa) to stimulate acupuncture points.

By taking these precautions, practitioners can increase the safety and efficacy of moxibustion therapy. These precautions include evaluating skin sensitivity and making sure the treatment area is properly ventilated to prevent smoke inhalation;

people with sensitive skin or a history of allergies should proceed cautiously or consult a healthcare provider before beginning moxibustion; practitioners should also be aware of fire safety protocols to prevent accidental burns or fires.

INCONSISTENCIES WITH SPECIFIC MEDICAL CONDITIONS

Patients with bleeding disorders or those who are prone to spontaneous bleeding should refrain from using moxibustion because it may increase the risk of bleeding. Moxibustion is contraindicated for people with specific medical conditions where the practice could potentially worsen their health. These conditions include fever, acute illness, or inflammation at the treatment site.

Patients who have cancer, especially those in areas that are receiving radiation therapy, should avoid having moxibustion on or near the affected regions to prevent negative reactions. Patients who are pregnant should consult with their healthcare providers before having moxibustion, as some acupuncture points may cause labor induction during pregnancy. Patients who have pacemakers or other electronic implants should also avoid having moxibustion near these devices to prevent interference.

SAFETY ADVICE FOR EXPECTANT MOTHERS AND KIDS

In particular, certain acupuncture points are contraindicated during pregnancy, especially those thought to stimulate uterine contractions or affect fetal development. Practitioners should modify treatment techniques to ensure safety and effectiveness while minimizing risks to mother and child. Pregnant women should consult with qualified practitioners familiar with prenatal acupuncture protocols.

Children's treatment sessions are usually shorter and use lower heat levels to prevent discomfort or adverse reactions; parents should communicate any concerns or observed reactions to the practitioner to ensure adjustments are made promptly; practitioners may also use alternative techniques like indirect moxibustion to enhance safety and comfort for pediatric patients. Moxibustion should only be performed under the supervision of experienced practitioners who understand pediatric acupuncture protocols.

TAKING CARE OF SMOKE AND ODOR ISSUES

Ventilation systems or open windows can help dissipate smoke quickly, reducing the risk of smoke inhalation and discomfort. Smoke and odor are common concerns during moxibustion therapy, particularly with direct burning of moxa. Proper ventilation is essential to minimize these effects, ensuring a comfortable environment for both the practitioner and the patient.

Indirect moxibustion techniques, like the use of moxa sticks or charcoal discs, can also reduce smoke production while delivering therapeutic benefits.

Patients with respiratory sensitivities or allergies should inform practitioners to enable adjustments in treatment methods or environments to effectively accommodate their needs. Practitioners should use high-quality moxa that produces minimal smoke and odor when burned, enhancing the treatment experience.

SOME ADVICE FOR REDUCING PAIN DURING MOXIBUSTION

Several useful suggestions and modifications to the treatment plan can help reduce discomfort during moxibustion. For example, making sure there is sufficient padding or insulation between the skin and the burning moxa can help prevent burns and direct heat exposure. Practitioners should also check in with patients to monitor their temperature and modify the intensity of treatment as needed.

Practitioners can incorporate brief intervals or breaks during treatment to allow the skin to cool down and minimize discomfort; patients should communicate any pain or discomfort immediately to their practitioner to ensure timely adjustments or cessation of treatment if necessary. Using smaller moxa cones or sticks allows precise application and reduces the risk of overheating sensitive areas.

CHAPTER EIGHT

FAQ CONCERNING MOXIBUSTION

WHAT AILMENTS ARE MOXIBUSTION CAPABLE OF CURING?

A popular traditional Chinese medicine treatment for pain management, moxibustion applies heat from burning moxa (dried mugwort) to specific acupuncture points or body regions to promote circulation and the flow of Qi (life energy) in the body's meridians. It is particularly useful for treating chronic pain conditions like arthritis and muscle stiffness. Additionally, by improving gastrointestinal function and regulating digestive processes, moxibustion can effectively treat digestive disorders like diarrhea and abdominal pain.

Additionally, moxibustion helps with gynecological problems like irregular periods and menstrual cramps. It works by balancing hormone levels and relieving menstrual discomfort by targeting acupuncture points related to reproductive health.

Moxibustion also helps with respiratory conditions like bronchitis and asthma because it boosts immunity and enhances respiratory function. Lastly, it helps with mental and emotional well-being by reducing stress, anxiety, and fatigue by calming and balancing the nervous system.

As a result of its ability to apply heat through the burning of moxa, moxibustion is a highly effective therapy for a variety of conditions, including pain management, digestive disorders, gynecological issues, respiratory conditions, and mental-emotional imbalances. Therefore, it is a valuable complementary treatment in holistic healthcare practices, as it stimulates circulation, enhances organ function, and balances the body's energy flow.

HOW FREQUENTLY SHOULD ONE ADMINISTER MOXIBUSTION THERAPY?

The number of moxibustion therapy sessions is determined by the patient's condition, health objectives, and a professional practitioner's recommendation. In general, moxibustion may be performed one to three times a week initially for chronic conditions that require ongoing management, such as digestive disorders or arthritis, to establish therapeutic benefits and gradually reduce symptoms over time.

Applying moxibustion more frequently, even daily if needed, can help with acute conditions or transient problems like a cold or strained muscle to speed up healing and reduce symptoms; however, the best frequency to use depends on the specific health needs and treatment objectives of each patient, so it's best to speak with a licensed acupuncturist or traditional Chinese medicine practitioner.

Moxibustion maintenance sessions may be suggested less regularly, such as once every 1-2 weeks or as needed, if desired changes in health or symptom relief have been achieved. This helps to maintain the therapeutic effects and avoid the long-term recurrence of problems.

The number of moxibustion therapy sessions varies based on the individual's health goals, the specific health condition, and the initial response to treatment. It is important to regularly consult with a qualified practitioner to ensure that moxibustion therapy is customized to meet the needs of each patient safely and effectively.

IS IT SAFE FOR ANYONE TO USE MOXIBUSTION?

When carried out by qualified professionals who follow the right procedures and hygienic guidelines, moxibustion is generally regarded as safe. However, there are some things to bear in mind about its safety for various populations.

It is important to consult with a healthcare provider or a licensed acupuncturist experienced in prenatal care to ensure the safety and appropriateness of moxibustion during pregnancy. Women who are pregnant should use caution when using moxibustion, especially avoiding specific acupuncture points that are contraindicated during pregnancy.

Practitioners frequently utilize protective barriers like ginger slices or salt cones to minimize direct skin contact and prevent unpleasant responses. People with sensitive skin, such as those with eczema, may experience skin discomfort from direct touch with burning moxa.

Moxibustion should be used with caution in individuals who have respiratory problems such as asthma, as the smoke released during the moxa-burning process may cause respiratory symptoms. To reduce these concerns, practitioners should use smokeless moxa or make sure there is enough ventilation during treatments.

Moxibustion is generally safe and well-tolerated; however, people should consult with qualified practitioners if they have any specific health concerns or conditions. Practitioners can customize moxibustion treatments to meet the needs and circumstances of each patient, ensuring safety and effectiveness.

WHAT IS THE WAY THAT MOXIBUSTION ENHANCES ACUPUNCTURE?

In traditional Chinese medicine, moxibustion and acupuncture are complementary therapies that are frequently combined to improve therapeutic results. Acupuncture stimulates the body's meridians and regulates Qi flow by inserting thin needles into specific acupuncture points; moxibustion applies heat to these points using burning moxa.

Combining acupuncture and moxibustion improves circulation, reduces pain, and improves overall health. Acupuncture needles stimulate nerve endings and improve Qi flow at acupuncture points, preparing them for the therapeutic heat of moxibustion.

The heat from moxibustion penetrates deeper layers of tissue, promoting relaxation of muscles and tendons, which can help to reduce pain and stiffness more effectively than acupuncture alone.

Moxibustion can also lengthen the duration of treatment benefits in addition to augmenting the effects of acupuncture.

Moreover, conditions made worse by cold weather or poor circulation benefit greatly from moxibustion's ability to warm the body and drive out cold. This complementary approach enables practitioners to tailor treatments according to the patient's constitution and particular health concerns, offering a comprehensive and integrated approach to healing.

Moxibustion is a complementary therapy that works in tandem with acupuncture to improve Qi circulation, reduce pain, and promote overall health and well-being. When combined, these therapies create a synergistic approach within traditional Chinese medicine that provides patients with comprehensive and individualized care that is customized to meet their specific health needs.

IS IT POSSIBLE TO SELF-ADMINISTER MOXIBUSTION AT HOME?

Self-administered moxibustion techniques typically involve using indirect methods to apply heat to acupuncture points or specific body areas. Although moxibustion is traditionally administered by trained practitioners, basic forms of moxibustion can be performed at home with appropriate guidance and precautions.

Using moxa sticks, which are essentially cigar-shaped rolls of moxa that may be lit and moved along meridians or across acupuncture sites, is one popular technique.

This indirect method minimizes direct skin contact with burning moxa, lowering the danger of burns or skin irritation.

Using a moxa box or burner, loose or cone-shaped moxa is placed on top of acupuncture points and burned until the heat from the moxa burns through the point, boosting Qi flow and encouraging therapeutic benefits. This is another way of indirect moxibustion.

Before attempting self-administration at home, people must receive proper instruction from a qualified practitioner regarding moxibustion techniques and safety precautions. Practitioners can offer guidance on the proper selection of moxa products, safe application of heat, and maintenance of adequate ventilation during treatments.

In conclusion, although indirect methods can be used to self-administer moxibustion at home, people should seek out appropriate instruction and guidance from qualified practitioners. If people take the necessary precautions and have the right knowledge, self-administered moxibustion can be a safe and effective addition to professional treatments, promoting overall health and well-being.

CHAPTER NINE

INCLUDING MOXIBUSTION IN YOUR DAILY ROUTINE FOR WELLNESS

HOW TO MAKE A CUSTOMIZED MOXIBUSTION SCHEDULE

Developing a customized moxibustion schedule entails figuring out your health objectives and incorporating moxibustion sessions in line with them. Start by determining your main areas of concern or where you hope to improve, like pain management, immunity building, or digestive issues. Then, research various moxibustion techniques, like direct or indirect moxibustion, and select the one that best suits your comfort level and medical requirements.

Next, create a regular schedule that works with your daily routine. This could involve scheduling moxibustion sessions at particular times of the day or week. Take into account factors such as the best time of day to focus on your health and relax, such as morning, afternoon, or evening.

Make sure your surroundings are safe and conducive to relaxation during moxibustion, including enough ventilation and a comfortable seating or lying position.

You can better adjust your schedule and techniques for best results by keeping a journal of your moxibustion sessions and their effects, including how long each session lasts, any sensations you experience during or after, and your overall feelings. You can also regularly review your progress and make necessary adjustments, such as adjusting the frequency of sessions based on your health goals and responses to moxibustion.

COMBINING MOXIBUSTION WITH ROUTINE SELF-CARE ACTIVITIES

By incorporating moxibustion into your regular self-care routine, you can increase its efficacy and make it a seamless part of your daily routine. To start, establish a relaxing routine around your moxibustion sessions.

You can prepare yourself for a more focused and beneficial moxibustion experience by using aromatherapy, relaxing music, or gentle stretching exercises.

Experiment with different combinations to find what works best for you in achieving a sense of holistic well-being. Moxibustion can be combined with other wellness practices like yoga, meditation, or tai chi to enhance its therapeutic effects. These practices complement moxibustion by promoting relaxation, improving circulation, and balancing energy flow throughout the body.

Consistency is key; aim to make moxibustion a regular part of your self-care routine to experience its cumulative benefits over time. After each moxibustion session, take some time to rest and hydrate to support your body's natural healing process. Notice any changes in your mood, energy levels, or physical symptoms, noting how moxibustion contributes to your overall well-being.

MONITORING DEVELOPMENTS AND HEALTH IMPROVEMENTS

A health journal or tracking app can be used to record daily or weekly changes in your symptoms and general well-being. First, set clear health goals that you hope to achieve with moxibustion, such as lowering pain levels, increasing digestive function, or improving sleep quality. Next, track your progress and monitor health improvements with moxibustion by methodically observing and documenting your body's responses to treatment.

During your moxibustion sessions, notice any immediate benefits you experience, such as warmth, increased relaxation, or altered perception of pain. Record these sensations, as well as any after-session benefits you receive. Then, over time, compare these observations to find patterns or trends in the ways that moxibustion influences your health outcomes.

This proactive approach enables you to optimize your moxibustion practice for customized health improvements. Regularly, review your tracking data to determine how well moxibustion is helping you achieve your health goals. Based on these insights, make necessary adjustments to your moxibustion schedule or techniques, seeking advice from a healthcare professional if needed.

SEEKING GUIDANCE FROM HEALTHCARE PROFESSIONALS

Seeking advice from medical professionals regarding moxibustion guarantees a safe and efficient incorporation into your wellness regimen. To find a qualified practitioner, look for one who specializes in acupuncture or traditional Chinese medicine, as these practitioners frequently possess knowledge of moxibustion techniques. Make an appointment to talk about your health objectives, existing medical conditions, and any worries you may have regarding moxibustion.

To determine whether moxibustion is appropriate for your particular health needs, the practitioner will perform a thorough assessment during the consultation. Depending on your condition, they may recommend specific techniques or modifications, ensuring individualized treatment that maximizes benefits and minimizes risks.

Maintain regular follow-up appointments to monitor progress and make further adjustments to your moxibustion plan as your health improves. Comply with the practitioner's recommendations for moxibustion sessions, including frequency, duration, and technique variations.

Be open and honest about your experiences and any changes in your health status to allow adjustments to be made as necessary for optimal outcomes.

EXAMINING MOXIBUSTION'S CULTURAL AND SPIRITUAL ASPECTS

Learn about the history of moxibustion in traditional Chinese medicine, its significance in Eastern health and wellness philosophies, and how it is perceived as a way to balance the body's energy (Qi) and promote harmony between the physical, mental, and spiritual dimensions.

These cultural and spiritual aspects of moxibustion will enhance your understanding and appreciation of this age-old healing technique.

Explore literature or teachings from various cultures that discuss moxibustion's role in maintaining health and preventing illness, offering insights into its broader implications beyond physical healing. Participate in cultural practices associated with moxibustion, such as ceremonies or rituals that honor its therapeutic benefits and historical legacy.

Consider your personal spiritual beliefs and how moxibustion fits into your journey toward wellness and self-discovery.

During moxibustion sessions, incorporate mindfulness or meditation practices to help you feel more connected to the healing process and inner peace. Moxibustion is a holistic approach to healing your body, mind, and spirit.

You can develop a greater understanding of moxibustion's therapeutic advantages and incorporate it into a comprehensive approach to well-being by investigating these cultural and spiritual aspects of the practice.

CHAPTER TEN

ADVANCED METHODS AND APPLICATIONS

USING MOXIBUSTION TO TREAT PERSISTENT PAIN

The use of mugwort (Artemisia vulgaris) burning over specific acupuncture points to promote circulation and reduce pain is known as moxibustion, a traditional Chinese medicine technique that has gained popularity in the treatment of chronic pain conditions. Moxibustion is particularly useful for treating areas where there is stagnation of qi or blood, which is thought to be the underlying cause of pain in traditional Chinese medicine theory.

The first step in the procedure is to identify the specific acupuncture points that correspond to the type and location of the pain. After that, the practitioner applies a small stick or cone of moxa directly to the skin or uses a moxa pole that hovers just above the skin's surface.

The moxa is lit and burns slowly, creating a deep heat that warms the surrounding tissues and the acupuncture point, stimulating circulation, relieving tension in the muscles, and encouraging the body's natural healing process.

Studies have shown that moxibustion is a useful treatment for several chronic pain conditions, such as arthritis, lower back pain, and menstrual cramps. It is frequently combined with acupuncture to improve treatment results. Patients who receive moxibustion therapy for chronic pain usually feel a slight warmth during treatment, and over several sessions, they may notice improvements in their mobility and degree of pain. Frequent sessions are advised for long-term pain relief and general health.

INNOVATIVE METHODS TO BOOST THERAPEUTIC IMPACT

The goal of advanced moxibustion therapy techniques is to maximize the therapeutic effects of the technique by improving application techniques and treatment protocols. One such technique is indirect moxibustion, which lowers the risk of burns while still providing therapeutic heat to the targeted area by holding the burning moxa slightly above the acupuncture point.

Utilizing smokeless moxa, which reduces smoke and odor during treatment and improves patient and practitioner comfort, is another method. Generally, smokeless moxa is made from mugwort and charcoal, offering a cleaner burning alternative without sacrificing therapeutic benefits.

In addition, practitioners can combine moxibustion with concurrent acupuncture to maximize the benefits of both therapies. This can improve pain relief and overall health by combining their advantages. Advanced practitioners frequently tailor treatment plans to the specific needs of each patient, modifying moxibustion techniques and frequencies to attain the best possible therapeutic results.

INCLUDING MOXIBUSTION IN SPORTS AND REHABILITATIVE MEDICINE

By incorporating moxibustion into sports medicine and rehabilitation, athletes and active individuals can benefit from a natural complement to traditional treatments for injuries and performance enhancement. Moxibustion targets specific acupuncture points associated with affected muscles and joints, reducing inflammation, improving circulation, and speeding up recovery. It can be used to relieve joint pain, muscle soreness, and stiffness that are frequently encountered during training or competition.

Athletes undergoing moxibustion therapy typically report faster recovery times and enhanced muscle flexibility, allowing them to return to peak performance sooner. In sports medicine, moxibustion is often integrated into comprehensive treatment plans alongside physiotherapy, massage, and stretching exercises. It can be especially helpful for chronic conditions like tendonitis or repetitive strain injuries, where conventional therapies may offer limited relief.

Integrative approaches that combine moxibustion with contemporary rehabilitation techniques show promise in optimizing recovery outcomes and supporting long-term athletic health.

Research into the application of moxibustion in sports medicine is still growing, with studies examining its effectiveness in treating sports-related injuries and enhancing athletic performance.

EXAMINING ADVANCES AND RESEARCH IN MOXIBUSTION THERAPY

To improve treatment outcomes and patient comfort, recent research and innovations in moxibustion therapy have focused on improving the therapy's efficacy, safety, and application across a range of health conditions. Examples of these innovations include smokeless moxa, adhesive moxa patches, and moxa poles that allow for precise control and application of heat.

Clinical trials have looked into how well moxibustion works to treat a variety of ailments, including nausea from chemotherapy, digestive issues, and even psychological issues like anxiety and depression.

It has been suggested that moxibustion may have therapeutic effects beyond pain management by modulating immune responses and neurotransmitters.

Other cutting-edge methods involve the integration of moxibustion with contemporary medical procedures, like mixing it with pharmaceutical treatments or physical rehabilitation programs.

This kind of interdisciplinary treatment seeks to maximize the benefits of both Western and traditional Chinese medicine to enhance patient outcomes and quality of life.

OPTIONS FOR MOXIBUSTION PRACTITIONERS' CERTIFICATION AND TRAINING

In nations where traditional Chinese medicine is recognized, moxibustion practitioners typically go through formal training that includes theoretical studies, practical skills in acupuncture and moxibustion techniques, and clinical experience under supervision. Certification and training options for moxibustion practitioners vary greatly depending on regional regulations and educational institutions.

Anatomy and physiology, theory of traditional Chinese medicine, acupuncture meridians, and specific moxibustion techniques are all covered in certification programs. Practical experience is necessary to become proficient in locating acupuncture points, applying moxa safely, and customizing treatments for each patient.

For moxibustion practitioners to remain current with advancements in the field, research findings, and changing clinical practices, they must pursue continuing education. Workshops, seminars, and online courses are frequently offered by professional organizations and associations, which also serve as a means of certification renewal.

To obtain certification, practitioners should confirm that the educational programs they are pursuing are accredited and that they are in compliance with any local laws that may regulate the practice of moxibustion. Ongoing professional development not only improves clinical skills but also cultivates a greater comprehension of the role that moxibustion plays in holistic healthcare approaches.

CHAPTER ELEVEN

UPCOMING DEVELOPMENTS AND TRENDS

NEW DEVELOPMENTS IN MOXIBUSTION DEVICES

The development of smokeless moxa devices, which eliminate the traditional smoke associated with burning moxa and use advanced heating elements to release therapeutic heat without combustion, is one notable innovation that has transformed traditional practices and made them more accessible and effective for modern users.

Another notable innovation is the rise in popularity of portable moxibustion kits, which enable practitioners to apply heat therapy conveniently at home or on the go.

These kits often include ergonomic designs and precise temperature controls, enhancing the user's ability to perform moxibustion with accuracy and comfort.

Digital moxibustion timers and controllers have made the practice easier by guaranteeing consistent treatment durations and temperature settings, thereby optimizing therapeutic outcomes and user experience. Another technological advancement in moxibustion devices is the incorporation of infrared heating technology. Infrared moxa lamps emit therapeutic infrared rays that penetrate deeply into tissues, promoting circulation and enhancing the therapeutic effects of moxibustion. This technology not only accelerates healing but also provides a non-invasive method for pain relief and relaxation.

The field of moxibustion is evolving along with technology, providing practitioners with cutting-edge tools that combine tradition and contemporary convenience.

These developments enhance the effectiveness of moxibustion therapy and make it more accessible to a wider range of people looking for natural healing alternatives.

RESEARCH ON MOXIBUSTION THERAPY TRENDS

Several studies have been conducted to investigate the mechanisms and benefits of moxibustion therapy in light of recent trends in the field. One area of particular interest is moxibustion's role in pain management and rehabilitation. Research has shown that moxibustion stimulates endorphin release and activates neural pathways involved in pain modulation, providing a non-pharmacological approach to pain relief. Researchers are also looking into moxibustion's potential to strengthen the body's defense mechanisms against infections and promote the production of anti-inflammatory cytokines, which in turn strengthens the body's natural defenses against infections.

A further developing trend is the integration of moxibustion with other complementary therapies, such as acupuncture and herbal medicine, to synergistically enhance treatment outcomes and address multifaceted health concerns.

Studies have suggested that moxibustion can reduce stress, anxiety, and depression in addition to improving mental health and overall emotional balance by regulating the autonomic nervous system and promoting relaxation responses.

Additionally, studies are examining tailored methods of moxibustion therapy, taking into account individual differences in response to care and refining protocols for particular medical conditions. These developments underscore the changing role of moxibustion in integrative medicine and present exciting directions for further investigation and practical applications.

VIEWS FROM AROUND THE WORLD ON TRADITIONAL CHINESE MEDICINE METHODS

Moxibustion is one of the many applications of traditional Chinese medicine (TCM) that have spread throughout the world due to its profound influence on health and wellness outside of East Asia. TCM has seen resurgence in popularity recently due to growing awareness of its holistic approach and success in treating chronic illnesses. Moxibustion has been adopted in particular because of its therapeutic benefits in boosting circulation, reducing pain, and reestablishing equilibrium in the body's energy systems.

TCM clinics that provide moxibustion services have multiplied in Western nations, serving a wide range of clients who are interested in complementary and alternative medicine. This widespread acceptance has encouraged partnerships between Western medical facilities and TCM practitioners to incorporate traditional therapies into mainstream healthcare settings. Additionally, professional associations and educational initiatives related to TCM have made knowledge-sharing and standardizing training programs for practitioners possible on a global scale.

Additionally, the UNESCO designation of moxibustion as an intangible cultural heritage has strengthened the practice's cultural significance and preservation efforts worldwide. As more people adopt TCM principles—including moxibustion—a growing trend is emerging that unites traditional wisdom with contemporary medical practices to promote a holistic approach to wellness that cuts across national boundaries.

SUSTAINABILITY OF THE ENVIRONMENT IN MOXIBUSTION MATERIALS

Concerns about deforestation and habitat loss have led to innovations in sustainable moxibustion materials, such as bamboo-derived moxa sticks and recycled packaging materials. Traditionally, moxa is derived from mugwort plants, which are cultivated using organic farming methods to minimize environmental impact and ensure purity. However, sustainability has become a focal point amid global efforts to promote eco-friendly practices in healthcare.

Additionally, efforts to preserve biodiversity and sustainable harvesting methods are crucial to preserving the ecological balance of the regions where moxibustion materials are sourced. Initiatives that support fair trade and ethical sourcing guarantee that local communities benefit from moxa cultivation while protecting cultural heritage and traditional knowledge. These developments in moxa production techniques also aim to lower carbon footprints and conserve natural resources.

Additionally, the use of biodegradable moxibustion accessories—like disposable ash catchers and natural fiber applicators—supports clinical and home waste reduction initiatives. These initiatives are in line with global sustainability goals and emphasize the significance of responsible production and consumption practices in the healthcare industry.

COMMUNITY SUPPORT AND EDUCATIONAL MATERIALS FOR MOXIBUSTION ENTHUSIASTS

Community support and educational resources are vital for developing moxibustion enthusiasts and encouraging safe, effective practices. Mobile applications and online platforms provide extensive instruction on moxibustion techniques, including video tutorials and interactive modules for both novice and seasoned practitioners. These resources cover important subjects like moxa selection, application techniques, and safety precautions, enabling users to advance their knowledge and abilities.

Social media groups and community forums allow moxibustion enthusiasts to connect with like-minded people around the world, exchange experiences, and seek advice. Peer-to-peer support networks facilitate learning and collaboration, promoting continued professional development and the sharing of best practices. Workshops and seminars led by seasoned practitioners and TCM experts offer practical training and continuing education credits, guaranteeing competency and proficiency in moxibustion therapy.

Furthermore, certification programs and licensure requirements validate competency and uphold quality assurance in moxibustion services, protecting patient safety and upholding professional integrity. Stakeholders also contribute to the growth and sustainability of moxibustion as a valued therapeutic modality in integrative healthcare by investing in education and community engagement. Professional associations and accreditation bodies are crucial in setting standards of practice and promoting ethical guidelines for moxibustion practitioners.